Copyright © 2021

Contents

What Is Microbiome Diet?

People tend to use the terms microbiome and microbiota interchangeably – but there is a distinct difference between the two. Microbiota (micro = tiny, biota = life) refers to the actual bacteria and other living microbes (yeasts, fungi, archaea) living in the gut (and other places on the body).

Microbiome, on the other hand, refers to the entire community or ecosystem of these microbes along with (as been suggested) their 'theatre of activity' AKA their genetic material, the environment they interact with (us!) and their physiological impact on their environment (us!).

The microbiome diet is a three-phase program that begins with an elimination diet, which claims to restore gut health in those who've been eating non-microbiome-friendly foods for a long time. Phases two and three are less restrictive, but all three phases focus on consuming mostly fruits, vegetables, lean protein, and a large amount of prebiotic and probiotic foods.

Foods that contain prebiotics and probiotics have risen to superfood status. You're probably familiar with probiotics and how they relate to gut health—there's hardly a health magazine that hasn't covered the topic. As "probiotics" and "gut health" became buzzwords during the mid-2010s, the 2014 publication of "The Microbiome

Diet" helped to popularize this style of eating and the myriad variations that followed.

Dr. Kellman research reveals that when the microbiome goes out of balance, people often gain weight, even when they haven't changed their diet or exercise. An imbalanced microbiome often dooms just about any diet to failure. When the microbiome is balanced, however, people often lose weight, even when they don't make any other changes.

Dr. Kellman posits that an imbalanced microbiome causes cravings for sugar and unhealthy fatty foods and that a balanced microbiome will increase your cravings for healthy foods. However, Dr. Kellman's diet may be missing a key element. Emerging evidence shows that it's not just bacteria that are crucial for gut health. The other microorganisms in the gut—particularly fungi—are just as important.

Learn how the microbiome diet works to determine whether it's a healthy choice for you.

How Does It Works?

There's no timing aspect to the microbiome diet. During all three phases of the plan, Dr. Kellman encourages intuitive eating, or eating when you're hungry and stopping when you're full. Those on this plan are also encouraged to avoid counting calories or tracking portions. This will help you learn to understand your body's natural hunger and satiety cues. The three phases of the diet are as follows:

Phase 1: The Four R's

The first phase of the microbiome diet is the most restrictive and is likely unnecessary for most people. During this 21-day phase, you're required to avoid a vast amount of healthy foods, including soy, dairy, grains, eggs, legumes, and starchy fruits, and vegetables. But you'll also cut out sugar and artificial sweeteners, packaged foods, fillers, or coloring, which can be a boon to your health.

The main foods encouraged in phase one are organic, prebiotic-rich foods, such as asparagus, garlic, leeks, and onions, and fermented foods such as sauerkraut and yogurt, which are rich in probiotics. Phase one is based on the "Four R's":

1. Remove: Eliminate any and all foods, chemicals, and toxins that may contribute to an unbalanced microbiome. This includes all processed foods, added sugar, hormones, antibiotics, and pesticides.

2. Repair: Consume large portions of plant-based foods and supplements to help heal the gut after years of harming it with processed foods and toxins.

3. Replace: Use herbs and spices and take supplements that can replace stomach acid and digestive enzymes to improve the quality of bacteria in your gut.

4. Reinoculate: Eat foods with high probiotic and prebiotic content to repopulate your gut with beneficial bacteria.

Phase 2: The Metabolic Boost

This 28-day phase allows for a little more flexibility based on the assumption that the first 21 days helped your gut grow stronger. Dairy, free-range eggs, legumes, and gluten-free grains can be added back into your diet during phase two. You can also start eating some starchy fruits and vegetables again, such as sweet potatoes and bananas.

During phase two, you still need to avoid certain foods about 90% of the time. This essentially means that you can have just a few servings a week of supposedly gut-damaging foods like soy, corn, and potatoes.

Phase 3: The Lifetime Tune-Up

By phase three, your gut should be fully "healed" or almost to that point, according to Dr. Kellman. Phase three is the maintenance phase of the microbiome diet, during which you can add back even more foods. The Lifetime Tune-Up is aptly named because followers of the microbiome diet are encouraged to maintain this style of eating for life.

Sample Microbiome Diet Food List

Each phase is a little different, but as a general rule, you're going to want to add foods that contain probiotics and prebiotics and avoid processed foods. Here are some of the foods you should and shouldn't eat once you've made it onto phase two:

What to Eat On the Microbiome Diet

- Non-starchy fruit and vegetables

- Lean protein

- Low-mercury fish

- Nuts and seeds (except peanuts)

- Prebiotic and probiotic foods

Foods to Avoid On the Microbiome Diet

- Packaged foods

- Grains and gluten

- Soy

- High fructose corn syrup and added sugars

- Artificial sweeteners

- Trans fats and hydrogenated oils

- Corn and potatoes

- Deli meat

- Peanuts

- Fried foods

- Fruit juice and dried fruit

- Starchy fruit and vegetables

- Eggs

- Dairy (except butter and ghee)

- Legumes (except chickpeas and lentils)

- Yeast and foods containing yeast

Non-Starchy Fruits and Vegetables

On the microbiome diet, you're encouraged to eat a substantial amount of berries, leafy greens, and other non-starchy produce, which is thought to have a variety of anti-inflammatory and antioxidant effects on the body.Non-starchy fruits include avocados, cherries, kiwi, citrus fruits, coconut, and tomatoes. Non-starchy vegetables include asparagus, artichokes, onions, radishes, and leeks.

Lean Protein

Almost all sources of animal protein are allowed on the microbiome diet, except eggs, which can be reintroduced later. Dr. Kellman encourages people to eat grass-fed meat. If you're choosing ground meats, look for ones with the lowest fat content possible.

Low-Mercury Fish

Mercury is toxic to humans, and like many health experts, Dr. Kellman recommends avoiding fish with high mercury levels. Low-mercury fish include salmon, trout, whitefish, mackerel, catfish, and sardines.

Nuts and Seeds

With the exception of peanuts (which are a type of legume), you can enjoy all kinds of nuts and seeds—and nut butters without added sugar—throughout the microbiome diet. Nuts and seeds are full of healthy fats, protein, and fiber that can help lower your cholesterol levels, aid in weight loss, and reduce inflammation.

Prebiotic and Probiotic Foods

These are the basis for the microbiome diet, and you should fill your diet with both prebiotic and probiotic foods. Prebiotics are a type of dietary fiber that provide food for the probiotic bacteria. Foods rich in prebiotics include artichokes, leeks, onions, dandelion greens, asparagus, and bananas—but remember that you can't eat bananas until phase two of the diet. Probiotic foods include kombucha, sauerkraut, pickles, tempeh, miso, kefir, and yogurt, but remember that soy and dairy aren't allowed during the first phase of the program.

Packaged Foods

Packaged foods are often full of fillers, additives, colorings, and chemicals, not to mention added sugar and sodium. Because packaged foods contain so many ingredients that may be harmful to the gut, they should be avoided at all times on the microbiome diet.

Grains and Gluten

Grains, especially those with gluten, are associated with inflammation in some people. You should avoid grains completely until phase two when you can reintroduce gluten-free grains such as quinoa and amaranth. You can start adding other whole grains back into your diet when you reach phase three, but Dr. Kellman advises that watch for any signs of intestinal discomfort.

Soy

Soy and soy products remain controversial. This is mostly because most soy is genetically modified and contains isoflavones, which led to the idea that soy causes breast cancer—though according to most studies, that isn't true. However, more recent evidence suggests that soy foods could actually have a beneficial effect on the gut microbiota. Whole soy products contain a good amount of prebiotic fiber.

High Fructose Corn Syrup and Added Sugars

HFCS or added sugars, in association with the standard American diet (high fat, high carbohydrate, and low fiber), may negatively alter gut microbes and cause cognitive issues, insulin resistance, and increase the risk for metabolic disease, inflammation, and inflammatory intentional disease.

Artificial Sweeteners

Some artificial sweeteners may alter the gut microbiome environment in both a positive and negative manner. However, the true mechanism of how artificial sweeteners interact with the human gut is not fully known. Further research is still needed.

Trans Fats and Hydrogenated Oils

Artificial trans fats and hydrogenated fats are made by pumping hydrogen molecules into vegetable oils, which turn the oil from a liquid at room temperature into a solid. Crisco, the popular baking ingredient, is a hydrogenated product. These kinds of fats can have detrimental effects on health and are associated with heart disease, diabetes, and arthritis. Trans fats also have a negative impact on gut bacteria and can result in dysbiosis (a microbial imbalance).

Corn and Potatoes

It's true that starchy foods can impact the composition of your gut microbiome. Many starches are resistant to digestion, which can alter the microbe environment. Not all starches have been tested, which is why it's recommended that you initially avoid corn, potatoes, and other starchy fruits and vegetables.

Deli Meat

Processed meat is to be avoided as fresh, lean meats are healthier alternatives.

Peanuts

Often mistaken for a tree nut, peanuts are actually legumes. Legumes are often shunned by many diet groups, including paleo followers. Peanuts are also a major allergen that can be adverse for many people. However, it's been found that peanuts might actually improve gut health in those who can tolerate them.

Fried Foods

You probably already know that fried foods aren't very good for you. The main reason for avoiding them is that they tend to reduce diversity in the gut bacteria. Generally, the more diverse your gut microbiome is, the healthier it is, too.

Fruit Juice and Dried Fruit

Fruit juice and dried fruit are to be avoided on the microbiome diet because they contain concentrated amounts of sugar.

Eggs

It's not eggs themselves that Dr. Kellman is concerned about—it's how they're produced. All eggs should be avoided until phase two, but when you add them back in, you should choose free-range, antibiotic-free eggs.

Dairy (Except Butter and Ghee)

Dairy, or rather the milk sugar lactose, is a common digestive irritant. Dr. Kellman recommends avoiding dairy with the exception of butter and ghee until phase two of the microbiome diet when you can begin eating probiotic-rich kefir and yogurt.

Legumes (Except Chickpeas and Lentils)

Legumes have a bad reputation when it comes to gut health, primarily because they contain lectins. Lectins are naturally occurring proteins in many foods, and they have been associated with inflammation and damage to the gut lining. But we know that legumes have many beneficial effects, too.

Yeast and Foods Containing Yeast

It's recommended that you avoid yeast on the microbiome diet because too much yeast consumption could lead to Candida overgrowth or other fungal infections in the gut.

Supplements to Take On the Microbiome Diet

Dr. Kellman recommends taking a handful of supplements on the microbiome diet in addition to focusing on gut-friendly foods. Here's a list of supplements to take while on the program:

• Berberine

- Caprylic acid

- Garlic

- Grapefruit seed extract

- Oregano oil

- Wormwood

- Zinc

- Carnosine

- DGL

- Glutamine

- Marshmallow

- N-acetyl glucosamine

- Quercetin

- Slippery elm

- Vitamin D

- Probiotic supplements

How does diet affect the microbiome?

We digest and absorb 80-95% of everything we eat and drink, but what's left travels through the large intestine where it interacts with the trillions of bacteria and other microbes that live there. So in thinking about nutrition, we have to think not only about how what we eat affects our bodies but also how it shapes the community of bacteria living within us.

The research has shown a number of observations on how human diet affects the gut microbiome:

- High saturated fat, high added sugar diets tend to create negative changes, favouring species such as Bacteroides

- High fibre diets tend to increase favourable species such as Lactobacillus and Bifidobacteriumand hinder the growth of less favourable species such as Clostridium

- Eating a diversity of plant foods is associated with improved diversity and resilience in the microbiome. According to findings from the American Gut Project, people more than 30 different plant foods a week is optimal.

- The gut microbiome can begin to change in as little as 24 hours in response to a major dietary shift

• Low FODMAP diets can reduce the overall size and diversity of the gut microbiota, which probably contributes to the effects of the diet and suggests that they not be long term

10 of the best foods for gut health

If you want to build a healthier gut, it's time to eat more plants! Whole plant foods offer an abundance of fibre, beneficial phytochemicals like polyphenols as well as a lower intake of added sugars and saturated fats. Moving towards a more anti-inflammatory, plant-rich diet will support your overall health and the health of your microbiome, as the research currently stands.

There is no need to be rigid in your eating habits: remember, it is what you do day in and day out that will determine your health more than what you put on a single plate. So have some ice cream once in a while, or a few fries.

And, if you're looking to supercharge your gut health, there are some foods that standout as anchors of a microbiome-friendly diet.

• Oatmeal + Barley

Oatmeal and barley are whole grains rich in soluble beta-glucan fibre. Beta-glucans have been shown to improve the growth of Lactobacillus and Bifidobacterium, two beneficial types of bacteria in the gut – along with improving the levels of short-chain fatty acids in the gut. Soluble fibre is also a great regulator of, ahem, elimination. Enjoy this yummy Pumpkin Spice Oats recipe.

- Berries

Berries such as raspberries and blackberries are super high in fibre, with raspberries containing 8g of fibre per cup. Blueberries and strawberries have slightly less (blueberries have 4g fibre per cup...still good!) but ALL berries are rich in polyphenols, a type of anti-inflammatory phytochemical that helps to boost beneficial bacteria and short-chain fatty acids in the large intestine.

- Turmeric

Turmeric is one of my favourite anti-inflammatory foods – it is polyphenol-rich and shown to improve markers of inflammation and even arthritis pain in early human trials. In lab and animal based trials, curcumin – the active component in turmeric – has been suggested to improve growth of beneficial gut bacteria and improve the barrier function of the gut. However, because human trials have yet to convincingly confirm lab results I recommend that people eat turmeric containing foods rather than supplements in most cases. Try this Turmeric Ginger Smoothie with Greens.

• Sunchokes (Jerusalem Artichokes)

Sunchokes – also known as fart-ichokes – are one of the highest sources of prebiotic inulin in the food supply. Prebiotics are substances known to improve the growth of beneficial bacteria in the gut. If you're new to prebiotics, start with a small amount to avoid tummy trouble.

• Sauerkraut + kimchi

Sauerkraut and kimchi are fermented foods that are typically made from a base of cabbage and other vegetables, along with salt to create a protective brine for fermentation. Lacto-fermented foods are rich in lactobacilli bacteria, making them a healthy addition to any digestive health eating plan – although they are not as potent as a clinical strength probiotic. I also like cabbage-based ferments as they are rich in l-glutamine, an amino acid that supports the health of the gut.

• Lentils + other legumes

Legumes are high fibre and high in prebiotic/FODMAP carbohydrates that feed beneficial bacteria in the gut. Eating legumes is associated with lowered risk of chronic diseases such as colorectal cancer. For those on a low FODMAP diet, you can still enjoy the benefits of small servings of lentils or chickpeas without triggering symptoms.

• Apples

Apples are one of the higher fibre fruits, while also having more soluble fibre (pectin) and prebiotic/FODMAP carbohydrates. They're affordable and available year round, so it's a great everyday gut health food.

• Ginger

This spicy cousin of turmeric is another one of my fave gut health foods. It is pro-kinetic, meaning it helps to improve stomach emptying and is often used for nausea in pregnancy.

• Leafy greens

Greens such as kale, spinach, chard and parsley are rich in fibre and anti-inflammatory polyphenols, both of which are fantastic for the gut. However, recently, it was also discovered that green leafy veggies contain a special sulfur-containing sugar called sulfoquinovose that drives the growth of beneficial E.coli in the gut (yes, some E.coli are good!).

• Garlic and Onions

Garlic and onions are rich in FODMAPs to feed beneficial bacteria in the gut – while garlic is also known to have antimicrobial properties that may support a healthy microbial balance. Interestingly, garlic and onions contain special sulfur-based phytochemicals such called glucosinolates which are thought to be anti-inflammatory when converted to isothiocyanate and early research is suggesting your gut bacteria may be capable of increasing the conversion.

Steps to a Healthier Microbiome

1. Eat a Plant-Based Diet with Lots of Fiber

The fiber in plant foods passes through the digestive system until it reaches the colon. Bacteria in the colon then break down the plant polysaccharides through fermentation into short-chain fatty acids, the largest amount as butyrate. Butyrate is the preferred energy source for cells in the colon and can help prevent colon cancer.

2. Eat Fermented Foods Every Day

Fermented foods, such as kimchi, sauerkraut, kefir, kombucha, tempeh, and miso all contain beneficial bacteria that can help fight against and crowd out the bad bacteria in your gut, resulting in a healthy balance of bacteria in the intestines. Aim for one to two servings of fermented food daily.

3. Consume Prebiotic-Rich Foods

Prebiotics, the preferred fuel source for your gut's good bacteria, is the indigestible fibers found in plant-based foods. Excellent sources of prebiotics include onions, garlic, artichokes, Jerusalem artichokes, jicama, green bananas, green banana flour, oatmeal, cooked and cooled rice and cooked and cooled potatoes.

4. Choose Polyphenol-Rich Foods

Polyphenols are micronutrients found in red wine, green tea, blueberries, pomegranates, cherries and dark chocolate that act as antioxidants. They decrease inflammation and stimulate the growth of beneficial bacteria while inhibiting the growth of pathogenic bacteria.

5. Take a Probiotic

Most probiotics contain various Lactobacillus and Bifidobacterium species. Another class of probiotics are soil-based organisms (SBOs), which have the ability to better survive the trip through the digestive system and reach the intestines intact, in order to "seed" the digestive tract with bacteria that will support a healthy microbiome. Opt for a probiotic with a large number of different strains.

6. Incorporate Collagen

Your hair, skin, nails and connective tissues are made of collagen. Collagen also acts as a protective covering for body organs like the kidneys. Unfortunately, aging, genetics, environmental pollutants and nutritional deficiencies deplete collagen. Adding it to your diet can help soothe and protect the gut lining and build new tissue.

7. Limit Sugar Intake

Sugar and artificial sweeteners feed the bad bacteria and can cause gastrointestinal distress in the forms of gas, bloating and diarrhea.

8. Be Mindful of Antibiotics

Antibiotics kill both the bad bacteria that make you sick and the good bacteria that keep you healthy. If you must take antibiotics for a bacterial infection, consider taking Saccharomyces boulardii, an antibiotic-resistant yeast that acts like a probiotic, as well as a multi-strain probiotic or a soil-based probiotic in between antibiotic doses. This will help repopulate good bacteria.

Pros and Cons

Pros

• Promotes nutritious food choices

• Improves gut health

• Limits sugar intake

Cons

- Restrictive

- Expensive

As with all diets, the microbiome diet has its benefits and drawbacks. Review the pros and cons to inform your decision about trying this eating plan.

Pros

- Promotes nutritious foods: The microbiome diet encourages people to choose whole, nutrient-dense foods such as fruit, berries, vegetables, fish, nuts and seeds, and lean protein. All of these food groups provide loads of vitamins and minerals, and they all have health-boosting properties.

- Improves gut health: More specifically, the fruits and veggies on the microbiome diet are gut-friendly foods. Asparagus, leeks, onions, artichokes, sauerkraut, kimchi, radishes, avocados, citrus fruits, and more all have prebiotic or probiotic qualities. Prebiotics and probiotics work together to achieve optimal gut health.

- Limits sugar intake: Excess sugar intake can be a driver of many chronic diseases and cause immediate symptoms such as lethargy, difficulty focusing, and mood swings. By limiting your sugar intake, the microbiome diet may help improve your day-to-day functioning.

Cons

- Restrictive: The microbiome diet can be very restrictive, especially in the first phase. It isn't usually necessary for most people to cut out as many foods as the first phase requires. Corn, soy, eggs, grains, legumes, and dairy can have a very healthy place in most people's diets.

- Expensive: The microbiome diet encourages organic foods, free-range meats, and cage-free eggs. These kinds of foods can be much more expensive than their traditional counterparts, so cost may be a limiting factor for many people on the microbiome diet.

Health Benefits

Health Maintenance

Research increasingly shows a strong link between a healthy diet and a healthy gut, and the link between a healthy gut and a generally healthy body.

Weight Loss

Because the microbiome diet requires you to eat mostly fruit, vegetables, and lean protein, it may inherently help you lose weight. Keep in mind, though, that it's still possible to take in more calories than you're burning even when you're eating healthy foods, which contributes to weight gain.

Disease Prevention

Some of the foods that have microbiome-friendly effects also have protective qualities against a number of diseases. For example, higher consumption of nuts and seeds has been associated with a reduced incidence of coronary heart disease, and gallstones (in both men and women), and diabetes in women. Limited evidence also suggests beneficial effects on hypertension, cancer, and inflammation.

Health Risks

Nutrient Imbalances

Phase one of the microbiome diet eliminates many healthy foods like whole grains, dairy products, eggs, starchy fruits and vegetables, and most legumes for 21 days. While these restrictions are temporary, they could result in nutrient imbalances.

Nutrition experts recommend skipping the first phase as it is unlikely that you need to cut out all of the foods it bans. Instead, it might be helpful to start with a more inclusive version, perhaps with the second phase. Even beginning with the third phase might be a big change for many people. For instance, if you currently eat a lot of artificial sweeteners, packaged foods, sodium, fried foods, and sugar, you could experience benefits just by following phase three of the microbiome diet, which is far more nutritionally balanced than phases one or two.

Disordered Eating

Some regimented diets with severe restrictions such as those found in phase one of the microbiome diet can lead to an unhealthy obsession with food. To that end, the microbiome diet may not be a healthy choice for those who have had or are at risk for developing an eating disorder.

Sample Microbiome Diet Meal Plan

Here is an example of a three-day meal plan on the first and strictest phase of the Microbiome Diet.

In phases two and three, your meal choices become increasingly more flexibility.

Day 1

- Breakfast: Fruit salad with Brazil nuts.

- Snack 1: Parsnip sticks with almond butter.

- Lunch: Chicken and vegetable soup.

- Snack 2: Roasted cauliflower with curry.

- Dinner: Grilled salmon with roasted Brussels sprouts, mixed greens, and fermented beets.

Day 2

- Breakfast: Pancakes made with almond flour topped with almond butter and fruit.

- Snack 1: Walnuts and cherries.

- Lunch: Vegetable salad topped with sauerkraut, chickpeas, and a parsley-lemon vinaigrette.

- Snack 2: Celery sticks with guacamole.

- Dinner: Zucchini noodles topped with marinara sauce and chicken meatballs.

Day 3

- Breakfast: Blueberry and almond breakfast cookies.

- Snack 1: Sautéed pineapple topped with shredded coconut.

- Lunch: Vegetable salad topped with miso-glazed cod.

- Snack 2: Carrots with hummus.

- Dinner: Flank steak tacos with steamed veggies, salsa, and guacamole.

MICROBIOME DIET RECIPES

Trying microbiome-friendly recipes is a great way to explore new flavors and find new favorite dishes while looking after your health. In this part are nourishing microbiome diet recipes for you to enjoy.

Baklava Butter

Preparation time

10 minutes

INGREDIENTS

- 1¼ cups walnuts

- 1/2 cup roasted almonds

- 1/3 cups pistachios

- 1/2 cup almond meal

- 1/4 cup organic honey

- 1 tablespoon coconut sugar

- 1 teaspoon ground cinnamon

- Pinch of sea salt

- 1 tablespoon extra-virgin olive oil

- 1 teaspoon vanilla extract

INSTRUCTIONS

1. In a food processor, combine the walnuts, almonds, and pistachios.

2. Pulse until coarsely ground or finely chopped—be careful not to over process.

3. Transfer the mixture to a medium bowl and stir in the almond meal.

4. In a small pot, combine the honey, sugar, cinnamon, and salt with 2 tablespoons of water.

5. Bring to a gentle simmer over low heat, then remove from the heat and add directly to the bowl with the nut mixture.

6. Add the olive oil and vanilla extract and mix well.

7. Transfer the butter to clean glass jar, refrigerate, and use within a week.

Berry-Kefir Smoothie

Preparation time

5 minutes

Ingredients

- 1 ½ cups frozen mixed berries

- 1 cup plain kefir

- ½ medium banana

- 2 teaspoons almond butter
- ½ teaspoon vanilla extract

Instructions

1. Combine berries, kefir, banana, almond butter and vanilla in a blender.

2. Blend until smooth.

Green Salad with Edamame & Beets

Preparation time

15 minutes

Ingredients

- 2 cups mixed salad greens

- 1 cup shelled edamame, thawed

- ½ medium raw beet, peeled and shredded (about 1/2 cup)

- 1 tablespoon plus 1 1/2 teaspoons red-wine vinegar

- 1 tablespoon chopped fresh cilantro

- 2 teaspoons extra-virgin olive oil

- Freshly ground pepper to taste

Instructions

1. Arrange greens, edamame and beet on a large plate. Whisk vinegar, cilantro, oil, salt and pepper in a small bowl. Drizzle over the salad and enjoy.

Avocado-Yogurt Dip

Preparation time

10 minutes

Ingredients

- 1 ripe avocado, peeled and pitted

- ½ cup nonfat plain yogurt

- ⅓ cup packed fresh cilantro leaves

- 2 tablespoons chopped onion

- 1 tablespoon lime juice

- ¼ teaspoon salt

- ¼ teaspoon freshly ground pepper

- Hot sauce to taste, optional

Instructions

1. Place avocado, yogurt, cilantro, onion, lime juice, salt and pepper in a food processor.

2. Process until smooth.

3. Season with hot sauce, if desired.

Kefir, banana, almond and frozen berry smoothie

Preparation time

10 minutes

Ingredients

- banana 1 ripe

- kefir 350ml

- mixed frozen berries 75g

- whole almonds 40g

- maple syrup or runny honey 1 tbsp

Instructions

1. Put everything into a blender or food processor and whizz until completely smooth.

2. Pour into 2 glasses and serve.

Miso salmon

Preparation time

35 minutes

Ingredients

- brown basmati rice 100g

- skinless salmon fillets 2

- pak choi 2, quartered lengthways
- sugar snap peas a handful

- baby corn a handful

- spring onions 2, thinly sliced

SAUCE

- white miso 1 tbsp

- rice vinegar 1 tbsp

- ginger a thumb-sized piece, finely grated

- garlic 1 clove, finely grated

Instructions

1. Cook the rice in lightly salted boiling water following pack instructions, then drain well.

2. For the sauce, whisk together all of the ingredients with 100ml of water.

3. Heat the grill to high and heat a non-stick oven-proof frying pan over a medium-high heat, lightly oil and season the salmon fillets then cook on one side for 2 minutes until crisp.

4. Turn, remove from the heat and pour over the miso sauce.

5. Put under the grill for 2-3 minutes or until the salmon is crisp and the sauce reduced and bubbling.

6. Meanwhile, cook the pak choi, sugar snaps and baby corn in a large pan of boiling water until just tender, then drain well.

7. Divide the rice and veg between two plates then add the salmon, spooning over any sauce.

8. Sprinkle with spring onions to serve.

Crispy spud salad with sauerkraut, ham hock and peas

Preparation time

1 hour

Ingredients

- new or Charlotte potatoes 400g, halved and large ones quartered

- spray oil

- smoked paprika 1 tsp

- lamb's lettuce 95g pack

- frozen peas 75g, defrosted

- sauerkraut 100g

- ham hock 90g pack

- flat-leaf parsley ½ a small bunch, chopped

DRESSING

- olive oil 1 tbsp

- Dijon mustard 2 tbsp

- white wine vinegar 2 tbsp

- caster sugar a pinch

Instructions

1. Heat the oven to 200C/fan 180C/gas 6.

2. Tip the new potatoes into a bowl and spray with oil, then add the smoked paprika and lots of seasoning.

3. Put onto a non-stick baking tray and roast for 40-45 minutes, turning halfway, until really golden.

4. Whisk together the dressing ingredients in a bowl then tip in the hot potatoes, lamb's lettuce and peas, and mix well.

5. Divide between 4 plates then top each with sauerkraut, ham hock and parsley.

kombucha

Preparation time

15 Minutes

Ingredients

- caster sugar 60g

- earl grey tea bags 3

- breakfast tea bags 2

- scoby 1, plus 100ml of kombucha liquid (this will come with the scoby when you order it)

Instructions

1. Put the sugar and 1 litre of just-boiled water into a pan and heat, stirring, until the sugar is dissolved.

2. Add the tea bags and leave to infuse for 5 minutes.

3. Carefully remove the teabags and leave the tea to cool completely.

4. Once cool, tip into a large glass jar with the scoby and kombucha liquid, cover the top with kitchen paper or muslin and seal in place with an elastic band or string.

5. Leave in a cool, dark place for 1-2 weeks, tasting daily after the first week – it should be funky and acidic but not overly sour.

6. Make sure you remove the scoby and 100ml of the liquid when you're happy with the final result.

7. Drink within a couple of days, keeping it in the fridge, or ferment a second time using the recipes below.

Kimchi-baked tofu

Preparation time

35 minutes

Ingredients

• firm tofu 280g block, cut into chunky pieces

• sesame seeds 2 tbsp, toasted

- long-stemmed broccoli 75g, halved horizontally

- sugar snap peas 75g

- baby sweetcorn 75g

- jasmine rice 100g

- spring onions 2, thinly sliced

- coriander a handful, leaves picked and stalks reserved

KIMCHI SAUCE

- kimchi 100g, drained

- ginger a thumb-sized piece, chopped

- garlic 2 cloves, chopped

- rice vinegar 1 tbsp

• soy sauce 1 tbsp

Instructions

1. Heat the oven to 200C/fan 180C/gas 6.

2. Put all the kimchi sauce ingredients and the coriander stalks into a blender or food processor and whizz until completely smooth, then pour in 75ml of water and whizz briefly again.

3. Pour into a small, deep baking dish and add the tofu pieces, tossing to coat.

4. Chill for 30 minutes.

5. Put the sesame seeds onto a plate then lift the tofu out of the marinade and roll in the seeds.

6. Put the broccoli, peas and corn into the baking dish, mix with the sauce then add the tofu on top.

7. Bake for 20 minutes until golden and the vegetables have cooked.

8. Meanwhile, put the rice, 200ml water and a pinch of salt into a small pan and bring to a simmer.

9. Put on a tight-fitting lid, turn the heat to low and cook gently for 10 minutes.

10. Remove from the heat and leave to steam with the lid on for another 10 minutes, then fluff up with a fork.

11. To serve, sprinkle over the spring onions and coriander leaves.

Sweet potato and miso mash

Preparation time

1 Hour 20 Minutes

Ingredients

• sweet potatoes 1kg

• white or red miso paste 1 1/2 tbsp

• butter 2 tbsp, plus a knob more

• vegetable stock 50-100ml, hot

• pumpkin seeds 2 tbsp

• lime zest to serve

• coriander leaves 2 tbsp, picked

Instructions

1. Heat the oven to 190C/fan 170C/gas 5.

2. Pierce the potatoes with a fork and bake for 50 minutes – 1 hour 10 minutes, depending on size, until they're really tender and a knife pokes in easily.

3. Halve the potatoes and spoon the flesh from the skins into a large pan.

4. Add the miso paste and butter and mash until really smooth.

5. Add the stock and mash again to get a spoonable consistency.

6. Taste if it needs any salt, reheat gently, then keep warm.

7. Fry the pumpkin seeds in a knob of butter in a small frying pan until hot and starting to toast or split.

8. Spoon the mash into a serving bowl, spoon the toasted seeds and butter over the top.

9. Season with freshly ground black pepper and a grating of lime zest, and scatter the coriander over to serve.

Cucumber kimchi

Preparation time

12 hours

Ingredients

- mini cucumbers 500g, halved lengthways

- flaky sea salt 2 tsp

- caster sugar 1 tsp

- apple ½, grated

- garlic 3 cloves, sliced

- ginger a thumb-sized piece, shredded

- gochugaru 2 tbsp, (see notes below)

- fish sauce 1 tbsp

- soy sauce 1 tbsp

- spring onions 3, shredded

Instructions

1. Put the cucumber pieces into a bowl and sprinkle over the salt.

2. Toss and leave for 20 minutes to draw out the moisture, then drain.

3. Put the sugar, apple, garlic, ginger, gochugaru, fish sauce and soy sauce into a bowl and mix well.

4. Add in the drained cucumbers and spring onions, and toss really well.

5. Spoon into a shallow dish and leave covered at room temperature for 12 hours or overnight, stirring every now and again.

6. It's then ready to serve or will keep covered in the fridge for a week, with the cucumbers becoming softer and funkier with time.

Prawn, cucumber and avocado salad with miso dressing

Prepartion time

15 Minutes

Ingredients

• white miso paste 3 tbsp

- rice wine vinegar 2 tbsp

- soy sauce 2 tsp

- sesame oil 1 tsp

- cucumber 1, seeded and cut into chunks

- radishes 200g, trimmed and quartered

- cooked peeled prawns 400g

- avocado 1, peeled, stoned and sliced

- salad leaves 100g

Instructions

1. Mix the miso, vinegar, soy sauce and sesame oil.

2. Whisk 1 tbsp water to loosen into a dressing.

3. Toss the cucumber, radishes and prawns with the dressing and gently fold in the avocado and salad leaves.

4. Tip onto a platter and drizzle over any remaining dressing.

Miso-buttered cod with broccoli, sesame and beans

Prepartion time

30 minutes

Ingredients

• miso soup sachet 1

• sesame oil 2 tsp

- Japanese rice vinegar 1 tbsp

- mirin 1 tbsp

- lime 1, juiced

- dried chilli flakes a couple of pinches

- tenderstem broccoli 8 spears

- spring onions 3, trimmed then thickly sliced

- green beans 100g, trimmed then thickly sliced

- edamame (soya beans) 150g, (see notes below)

- unsalted butter 2 tsp, softened

- brown miso 1 tbsp

- sesame seeds (black, white or a mixture) or furikake seasoning 1 tbsp, (see notes below)

- chunky cod fillets 2

Instructions

1. Heat the oven to 200C/fan 180C/gas 6.

2. Empty the miso soup sachet into a jug and top up with 400ml of boiling water.

3. Stir in the sesame oil, vinegar, mirin, lime juice and chilli flakes.

4. In a deep roasting tin (about 20 x 30cm), group together the broccoli to make two rafts for the fish.

5. Scatter the rest of the green veg around and pour over the miso stock.

6. Mash together the butter, brown miso and sesame seeds or furikake with some pepper.

7. Spread 1/2 over the top of each cod fillet, then sit each on top of a broccoli raft.

8. Roast for 20 minutes until the cod flesh is just flaking, and the veg is just cooked but still a little crunchy.

Confit garlic with roasted tomatoes on toast

Preparation time

1 hour 15 minutes

Ingredients

- garlic 4 whole bulbs

- thyme 6 sprigs

• olive oil 400ml

• cherry tomatoes 300g, halved

• sourdough 4 slices, toasted

Instructions

1. Heat the oven to 160C/fan 140C/gas 3.

2. Cut the garlic bulbs horizontally across the tops, so that all of the cloves are revealed, and sit them snugly into a small, deep roasting tin.

3. Add the thyme sprigs and a generous pinch of salt, and pour over the oil until the bulbs are nearly submerged, adding a little more if needed.

4. Cook for an hour or until the cloves are really soft.

5. Put the cherry tomatoes cut-side up into a roasting tin and sprinkle with salt.

6. Put into the oven for the final 25 minutes of the garlic's cooking time.

7. Use a spatula to lift the garlic bulbs from the oil and cool slightly.

8. Squeeze the cloves from their skins onto the toasted sourdough and pile on the tomatoes, along with a little of the garlic-perfumed oil (keep the rest for cooking – it will keep for two weeks in the fridge).

Broccoli and blue cheese salad

Preparation time

20 minutes

Ingredients

• purple sprouting broccoli 400g, trimmed

• olive oil 1 tbsp, plus extra to serve

• lemon ½, juiced

• blanched almonds 100g, toasted and roughly chopped

DRESSING

- olive oil 1 tbsp

- garlic 1 small clove, sliced

- blue cheese 100g, crumbled

- lemon ½, zested and juiced

- natural yogurt 30g

- chives a small bunch, finely chopped

Instructions

1. Bring a large pan of salted water to the boil.

2. Cook the broccoli for 2 minutes until tender, drain well and tip into a bowl with the olive oil and lemon juice.

3. Cool completely.

4. To make the dressing, fry the garlic with the olive oil in a pan for 2 minutes.

5. Put the rest of the dressing ingredients into a blender along with the fried garlic and oil, and season generously.

6. Whizz until completely smooth, adding 1-2 tbsp of water if it's a little thick.

7. To finish, put the broccoli on a serving plate and drizzle generously with the dressing and a splash of olive oil followed by the chopped almonds.

Broccoli tabouli with feta and pomegranate

Preparation time

20 minutes

INGREDIENTS

- 350g broccoli, cut into florets

- 4 green shallots, thinly sliced

- 400g can chickpeas, rinsed, drained

- 1 Lebanese cucumber, coarsely chopped

- 200g mixed grape tomatoes, halved

- 1/2 cup fresh mint leaves, finely chopped

- 2 cups fresh continental parsley leaves, finely chopped

- 1 lemon, juiced

- 2 tbs pomegranate molasses

- 40g (1/4 cup) marinated feta, crumbled

- 1 tablespoon pine nuts, toasted

- Pomegranate seeds, to serve (optional)

- Lemon wedges, to serve

Instructions

1. Process the broccoli in a food processor until it's finely chopped and resembles rice.

2. Combine broccoli, shallot, chickpeas, cucumber, tomato, mint and parsley in a large bowl. Season.

3. Toss to combine.

4. Place the lemon juice and pomegranate molasses in a small jug and whisk to combine. Season.

5. Pour over the tabouli and toss to combine.

6. Transfer the tabouli to a large serving platter.

7. Top with the crumbled marinated feta, toasted pine nuts and pomegranate seeds, if using.

8. Serve with lemon wedges.

Honey soy tempeh with udon

Prepartion time

17 minutes

INGREDIENTS

- 300g tempeh, sliced

- 2 garlic cloves, crushed

- 60ml (1/4 cup) store-bought honey and soy marinade

- 2 teaspoon sesame oil

- 2 bunches broccolini, trimmed, sliced

- 120g baby kale

- 180g Hakubaku Udon Noodles

- 45g (1/4 cup) tamari almonds, coarsely chopped

- Sriracha chilli sauce, to serve

Instructions

1. Combine the tempeh, garlic, 1 tablespoon honey and soy marinade and 1 teaspoon sesame oil in a bowl.

2. Heat a large wok or non-stick frying pan over medium-high heat.

3. Add remaining 1 teaspoon sesame oil and swirl to coat the base.

4. Add the broccolini and stir-fry for 1-2 minutes or until just tender but still crisp.

5. Add the kale and stir-fry for 1 minute or until wilted.

6. Transfer to a plate and cover to keep warm.

7. Cook the noodles in a large saucepan of boiling water following packet directions. Drain.

8. Meanwhile, spray the wok with oil. Cook tempeh, in 2 batches, for 1-2 minutes each side or until golden and lightly caramelised.

9. Divide the noodles among serving bowls.

10. Top with the tempeh and the broccolini mixture.

11. Drizzle with the remaining 2 tbs honey and soy marinade.

12. Sprinkle with almonds and serve drizzled with chilli sauce.

Smoothie bowl

Preparation time

15 minutes

INGREDIENTS

- 20g (1/4 cup) shredded coconut

- 2 tablespoons raw buckwheat

- 2 tablespoons pepitas

- 2 bananas, coarsely chopped
- 50g (1/2 cup) rolled oats

- 150g (1 cup) frozen berries, plus extra, to serve

- 70g (1/4 cup) Vaalia natural yoghurt, plus extra to swirl

- 2 tablespoons vanilla protein powder

- 375ml (1 1/2 cups) milk

- Raw cacao nibs, to serve

- Chia seeds, to serve

Instructions

1. Preheat oven to 200C/180C fan forced.

2. Line a baking tray with baking paper.

3. Place the coconut, buckwheat and pepitas on the prepared tray.

4. Bake for 5-10 minutes or until golden.

5. Set aside to cool.

6. Blend bananas, oats, berries, yoghurt, protein powder and milk in a blender until smooth.

7. Divide among bowls.

8. Swirl in extra yoghurt and top with cacao, chia and extra berries.

Lemon Chicken Stew (altered)

Microbiome Diet

Prepartion time

1 hour

INGREDIENTS

- 1 unit (yield from 1 lb ready-to Chicken Thigh

- 2 tbsp Olive Oil

- .5 cup, chopped Onions, raw

- 1 cup, strips or slices Carrots, raw

- 1 cup slices Parsnips

- 2 clove Garlic

- 2 serving Lemon, fresh squeezed, juice of one whole lemon

- 2 serving Pacific Natural Foods Organic Free Range Chicken Broth, 1 cup

- .5 tbsp Rosemary

- 1 tsp Thyme, ground

- 5 cup Jerusalem Artichoke (Sunchoke) (by DHARMAHEART)

- 1 stalk, large (11"-12" long) Celery, raw

- 1 tbsp Parsley

- 5 cup Spinach, fresh

Instructions

1. Preheat oven to 350. Saute chicken in 1 tbsp olive oil, on med-high, until lightly browned, about 10 minutes.

2. Transfer chicken to baking pan.

3. Add remaining oil, onion, and celery until soft.

4. Add carrot, sunchoke, and parsnip to saute pan, and cook for 5 minutes on med-high heat until lightly browned.

5. Add lemon juice/zest garlic, chicken broth chopped rosemary, thyme, chopped spinach, and parsley.

6. Cook for 5 minutes.

7. Pour mixture over chicken, and cover baking pan with foil. Bake for 30 minutes, or until tender.

8. Salt and pepper to taste, and top with rosemary sprigs(optional).

Veggie Niçoise Salad with Red Curry Green Beans

Preparation time

1 hour

INGREDIENTS

DRESSING

- 1 large shallot, minced

- 1 garlic clove, minced

- 1 tablespoon Dijon mustard

- 3 tablespoons white wine vinegar

- ½ cup extra-virgin olive oil

- Kosher salt

- Freshly ground black pepper

SALAD

- ¾ pound new potatoes

- 2 tablespoons white wine vinegar

- 2 tablespoons extra-virgin olive oil

- ½ tablespoon red curry paste

- ½ pound green beans, trimmed

- Kosher salt

- Freshly ground black pepper

- 4 cups baby arugula

- 1 bunch radishes, quartered

- ½ English cucumber, thinly sliced

- 3 large hard-boiled eggs, halved lengthwise

- 1 cup halved Niçoise olives

Instructions

1. MAKE THE DRESSING: In a small bowl, whisk together the shallots, garlic, mustard and vinegar. Gradually whisk in the oil until the mixture is thick.

2. Season with salt and pepper.

3. MAKE THE SALAD: In a large pot, cover the potatoes with 1 inch of water and bring to a boil. Cook until the potatoes are fork-tender, 8 to 10 minutes.

4. Drain and cool slightly.

5. Meanwhile, in a medium bowl, whisk together the vinegar, olive oil and curry paste.

6. Add the green beans and toss well to coat.

7. Season with salt and pepper.

8. In a large bowl, toss the arugula with half of the dressing and then transfer to a large platter.

9. In three separate small bowls, toss the potatoes, radishes and cucumber slices with the remaining dressing.

10. Top the arugula with the potatoes, green beans, radishes, cucumber, hard-boiled eggs and olives.

Cauliflower Steaks with Lemon-Herb Sauce

Preparation time

45 minutes

INGREDIENTS

LEMON-HERB SAUCE

- 1 cup parsley leaves

- ½ cup cilantro leaves

- ½ cup mint leaves

- ½ cup roughly chopped green onion

- 1 garlic clove, smashed

* Juice of 1 lemon

* ⅓ cup olive oil

CAULIFLOWER STEAKS

* 1 large head cauliflower

* 4 tablespoons extra-virgin olive oil, divided

* 4 teaspoons smoked paprika

* Salt and freshly ground black pepper, to taste

Instructions

1. MAKE THE HERB SAUCE: In a blender or food processor, pulse the parsley, cilantro, mint, green onion, garlic, lemon juice and olive oil until completely smooth. Set aside.

2. MAKE THE CAULIFLOWER STEAKS: With a sharp knife, cut the cauliflower into 1-inch-thick slices. (You should get about 8 slices.) Rub both sides of each piece of cauliflower with about 1 teaspoon olive oil. Sprinkle both sides of each piece with ½ teaspoon smoked paprika, salt and pepper.

3. Heat the remaining 1 tablespoon olive oil in a large cast-iron skillet over medium-high heat. Working in batches, sear the cauliflower steaks until they are golden brown, 3 to 4 minutes per side. The cauliflower should be easily pierced with a fork but not so tender that it falls apart.

4. To serve, place 2 cauliflower steaks on each plate and top with a generous drizzle of the lemon-herb sauce. Serve immediately.

Spicy Carrot Salad with Chickpeas and Parsley

Preparation time

20 minutes

INGREDIENTS

SALAD

- 3 large carrots--washed, dried and ends trimmed

- One 14.5-ounce can chickpeas, drained

- 1 cup parsley leaves, loosely packed

DRESSING

- ⅓ cup extra-virgin olive oil

- 3 tablespoons harissa

- 1 tablespoon white-wine vinegar

- 1 lemon, zested and juiced

- 1 teaspoon ground cumin

- Salt and freshly ground black pepper

Instructions

1. MAKE THE SALAD: Shred the carrots using a box grater (as if you're making coleslaw).

2. Transfer the shredded carrots to a large bowl and toss with the chickpeas and parsley leaves.

3. MAKE THE DRESSING: In a small bowl, whisk the olive oil with the harissa to combine.

4. Slowly add the vinegar and lemon juice.

5. Stir in the lemon zest and cumin, then season with salt and pepper.

6. Add the salad dressing to the carrot mixture and toss to coat.

7. Serve at room temperature or chilled (it will keep in the fridge for up to three days in an airtight container).

COCONUT AND GINGER PUMPKIN SOUP

Preparation time

55 minutes

Ingredients

- 1 kilogram pumpkin – any variety will do, I used Kent pumpkin for the soup pictured

- 500 mL chicken broth or stock – substitute vegetable stock for a vegan/vegetarian soup

- 250 mL coconut milk

- 60 grams fresh ginger (about 3-4 thumb sized pieces)

- 1 tsp ground cumin

- 1/2 tsp ground cinnamon

- 2 tbsp extra virgin olive oil for roasting the pumpkin – can also use coconut oil

• salt and pepper to taste

Ingredients

1. Preheat oven to 180 C and line a large tray with baking paper (or use a non-stick tray).

2. Peel pumpkin and cut into even-sized chunks.

3. Place on tray, drizzle over olive oil and toss around with your hands to coat.

4. Roast pumpkin in the oven for approximately 45 minutes or until super soft and starting to caramelize at the edges.

5. While the pumpkin is roasting, peel the ginger and gather the rest of the ingredients.

6. Place cooked pumpkin, chicken broth/stock, coconut milk, ginger, cumin and cinnamon into blender jug.

7. Blend until super smooth.

8. Season with salt and pepper to taste.

9. To serve, heat a portion of the soup in a saucepan over the stove (or microwave the soup if that's more convenient for you). Enjoy!

Baddha Bowl with Kale, Avocado, Orange and wild Rice

Preparation time

40 minutes

INGREDIENTS

RICE

- 1 cup wild rice

- 3 cups vegetable broth or water

- 1 garlic clove, minced

- 2 tablespoons extra-virgin olive oil

- 2 tablespoons rice vinegar

- 1 tablespoon chopped fresh mint

- Salt and freshly ground black pepper

TOPPINGS

- 1 bunch kale, roughly chopped

- 2 tablespoons olive oil

- 1 tablespoon rice vinegar

- ¼ cup pomegranate seeds

- 1 orange, cut into segments

- ½ avocado, sliced

- ¼ cup pumpkin seeds

- 2 hard-boiled eggs

- Salt and freshly ground black pepper

Ingredients

MAKE THE RICE: In a medium pot, stir the rice with the broth (or water, if using) and garlic to combine. Bring the mixture to a simmer over medium-high heat.

Once the liquid is boiling, reduce the heat to low and simmer until the rice is tender and all the liquid has been absorbed, 15 to 17 minutes.

Let the rice cool for 5 to 10 minutes and then toss it with the olive oil, vinegar, mint, salt and pepper.

MAKE THE TOPPINGS: In a medium bowl, toss the kale with the olive oil and vinegar.

Divide the rice between two bowls and then top with equal amounts of kale.

Top each of the bowls with 2 tablespoons pomegranate seeds, half the orange slices, half the avocado slices, 2 tablespoons pumpkin seeds and a hard-boiled egg.

Season the egg with salt and pepper.

Serve immediately.

Whole30 Chicken Meatballs and Cauliflower Rice with Coconut-Herb Sauce

Preparation time

50 minutes

INGREDIENTS

MEATBALLS

- Nonstick spray

- 1 tablespoon extra-virgin olive oil

- ½ red onion

- 2 garlic cloves, minced

- 1 pound ground chicken

- ¼ cup chopped fresh parsley

- 1 tablespoon Dijon mustard

- ¾ teaspoon kosher salt

- ½ teaspoon freshly ground black pepper

SAUCE

- One 14-ounce can coconut milk

- 1¼ cups chopped fresh parsley, divided

- 4 scallions, roughly chopped

- 1 garlic clove, peeled and smashed

- Zest and juice of 1 lemon

- Kosher salt and freshly ground black pepper

- Red pepper flakes, for serving

- 1 recipe Cauliflower Rice

Instructions

MAKE THE MEATBALLS:

1. Preheat the oven to 375°F.

2. Line a baking sheet with aluminum foil and spray it with nonstick spray.

3. In a medium skillet pan, heat the olive oil over medium heat. Add the onion and sauté until tender, about 5 minutes.

4. Add the garlic and sauté until fragrant, about 1 minute.

5. Transfer the onion and garlic to a medium bowl and cool slightly.

6. Stir in the chicken, parsley and mustard; season with salt and pepper.

7. Form the mixture into 2 tablespoon-size balls and transfer to the baking sheet.

8. Bake the meatballs until firm and fully cooked, 17 to 20 minutes.

MAKE THE SAUCE:

1. In the bowl of a food processor, combine the coconut milk, parsley, scallions, garlic, lemon zest and lemon juice and process until smooth;

2. season with salt and pepper.

3. Top the meatballs with the red pepper flakes and the remaining parsley.

4. Serve over the cauliflower rice with the sauce.

Egg and Veggie Breakfast Bowl

Prepartion time

35 minutes

INGREDIENTS

1 pound Brussels sprouts

1 pound sweet potatoes

1½ tablespoons olive oil

2 cups arugula

4 eggs

2 tablespoon harissa

3 tablespoons apple cider vinegar

Instructions

1. Preheat the oven to 400°F.

2. Line a baking sheet with parchment paper.

3. Cut the Brussels sprouts in half.

4. Dice the sweet potatoes.

5. Spread out the brussels sprouts and sweet potatoes on the baking sheet. Drizzle the olive oil evenly over the vegetables; season with salt and pepper.

6. Roast in the oven until golden brown and tender, 17 to 20 minutes.

7. In a small bowl, whisk the harissa with the olive oil and apple cider vinegar.

8. Poach or fry the eggs. (Need a little help? Here's a tutorial on how to poach, and here's a tutorial on how to fry.)

9. To serve, divide the brussels sprouts and sweet potatoes among four bowls; top each with ½ cup arugula and 1 egg.

10. Drizzle each bowl with 2 teaspoons of the harissa vinaigrette.

PINEAPPLE MANGO SALSA CHICKEN LETTUCE WRAPS

Preparation time

20 minutes

Ingredients

- 2 cups shredded chicken (approx 1 lb)

- 1 tablespoon olive oil

- 1/2 teaspoon paprika

- 1 tablespoon lime juice

- 1/2 teaspoon garlic powder

- 1/4 teaspoon salt

- 1 cup Pineapple Mango Salsa

- 10 lettuce wraps (romaine lettuce)

Instructions

1. Follow this recipe for 10 minute shredded chicken in the instant pot. If you don't have an instant pot, bring a pot of water to a boil and boil chicken on the stove for 10 minutes. Otherwise, use rotisserie chicken.

2. While chicken is cooking, assemble Pineapple Mango Salsa.

3. Toss cooked, shredded chicken with olive oil, paprika, garlic powder, salt and lime juice

4. Assemble lettuce wraps layering chicken + salsa.

5. Top with avocado or additional lime juice for flavor.

One - Pan Roasted Salmon with Potatoes and

Romaine

Preparation time

40 minutes

INGREDIENTS

• 1 pound baby Yukon Gold potatoes (or another bite-sized potato)

• 4 tablespoons extra-virgin olive oil, divided

- 1 teaspoon lemon juice

- Kosher salt and freshly ground black pepper, to taste

- Four 6-ounce salmon fillets

- 1 tablespoon unsalted butter, melted

- ¼ teaspoon paprika

- 2 hearts romaine lettuce

Instructions

1. Preheat the oven to 400°F.

2. In a medium bowl, toss the potatoes with 2 tablespoons of the olive oil; arrange in a single layer on a baking sheet.

3.   Roast the potatoes in the oven until slightly golden and fork-tender, 15 to 20 minutes.

4. Meanwhile, cut the romaine hearts in half and rub with 2 tablespoons olive oil and the lemon juice. Season with salt and pepper. Set aside.

5. Using a pastry brush, brush the salmon fillets with the melted butter.

6. Season each fillet with paprika and salt and pepper to taste.

7. Arrange the romaine hearts and salmon on the baking sheet with the potatoes.

8. Continue roasting until the lettuce is tender and the fish is cooked through, 5 to 7 minutes more.

9. To serve, divide the potatoes, romaine and salmon among four plates.

Sweet Potato Protein Breakfast Bowl

Preparation time

5 minutes

INGREDIENTS

- 1 small sweet potato, pre-baked

- 1 serving protein powder*

- 1 small banana, sliced

- 1/4 cup raspberries
- 1/4 cup blueberries

optional toppings

- cacao nibs

- chia seeds

- hemp hearts

- favorite nut/seed butter

INSTRUCTIONS

1. Flesh out sweet potato if not done already.

2. In a small bowl, mash sweet potato with fork.

3. Stir in protein powder until combined.

4. Layer in banana slices, raspberries, and blueberries.

5. Top with additional desired toppings and dig in! You can enjoy this bowl warm or cold, your choice!

Cauliflower Fried Rice

Preparation time

25 minutes

Ingredients

FRIED RICE

• 1 head cauliflower, cut into florets

• 2 tablespoons neutral oil (such as vegetable, coconut or peanut)

• 1 bunch scallions, thinly sliced

- 3 garlic cloves, minced

- 1 tablespoon minced fresh ginger

- 2 carrots, peeled and diced

- 2 celery stalks, diced

- 1 red bell pepper, diced

- 1 cup frozen peas

- 2 tablespoons rice vinegar

- 3 tablespoons soy sauce

- 2 teaspoons Sriracha, or more to taste

GARNISHES

- 1 tablespoon neutral oil (such as vegetable, coconut or peanut)

- 4 eggs

- Salt and freshly ground black pepper

- 4 tablespoons chopped fresh cilantro

- 4 tablespoons thinly sliced scallions

- 4 teaspoons sesame seeds

Instructions

MAKE THE FRIED RICE:

1. In the bowl of a food processor, pulse the cauliflower until the mixture resembles rice, 2 to 3 minutes. Set aside.

2. In a large skillet, heat the oil over medium heat.

3. Add the scallions, garlic and ginger, and stir-fry until fragrant, about 1 minute.

4. Add the carrots, celery and red bell pepper, and stir-fry until the vegetables are tender, 9 to 11 minutes.

5. Add the cauliflower rice and stir-fry until it begins to turn golden, 3 to 5 minutes more.

6. Stir in the frozen peas and toss well to combine.

7. Add the rice vinegar, soy sauce and Sriracha, and toss to combine. Set aside.

MAKE THE GARNISHES:

1. In a medium skillet, heat the oil over medium-high heat.

2. Crack the eggs directly into the pan and cook until the whites are set but the yolks are still runny, 3 to 4 minutes.

3. Season each with salt and pepper.

4. To serve, divide the cauliflower rice among four plates and top each with a fried egg.

5. Garnish each plate with 1 tablespoon cilantro, 1 tablespoon scallions and 1 teaspoon sesame seeds.

6. Serve immediately.

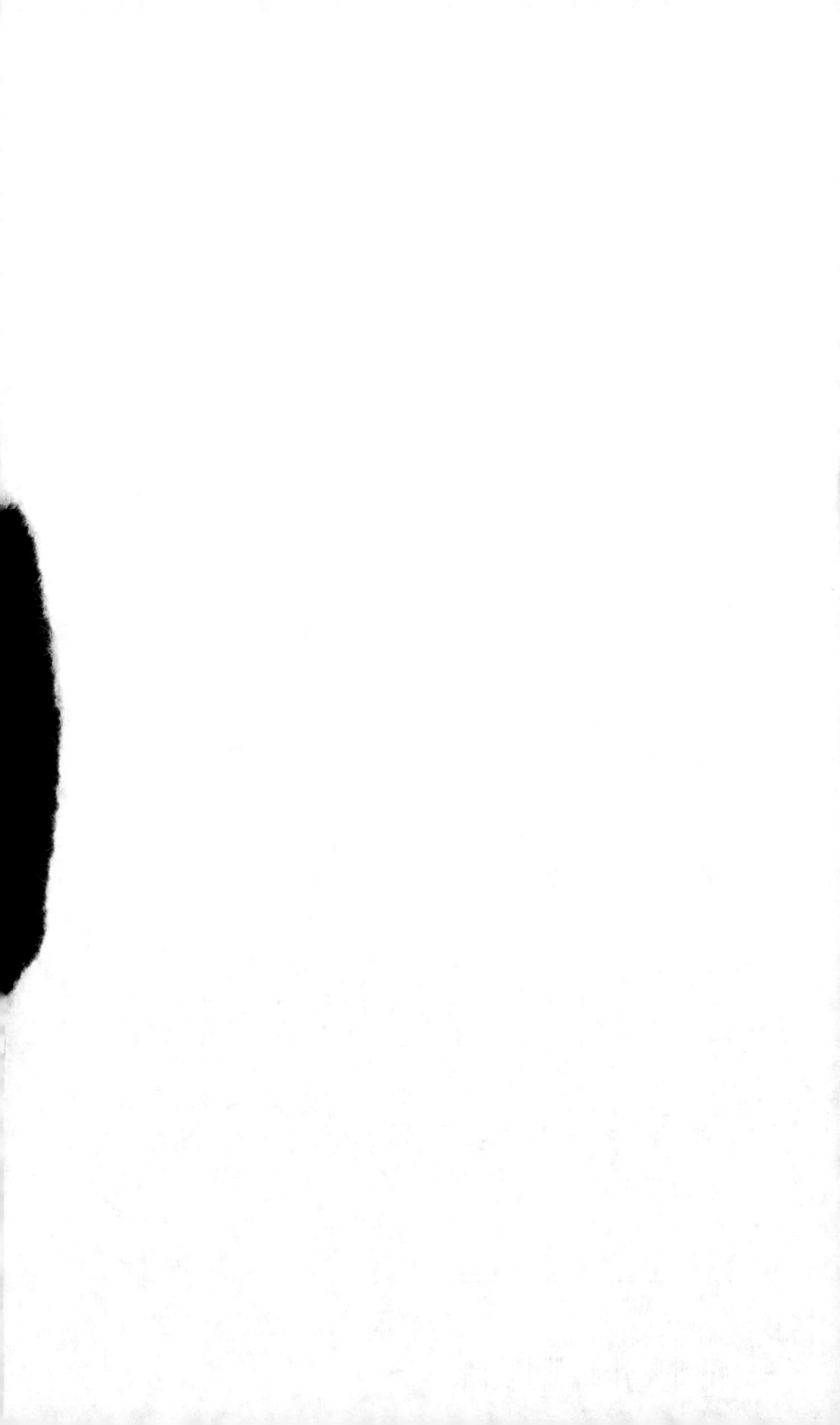